YOUR KNOWLEDGE HAS VALUE

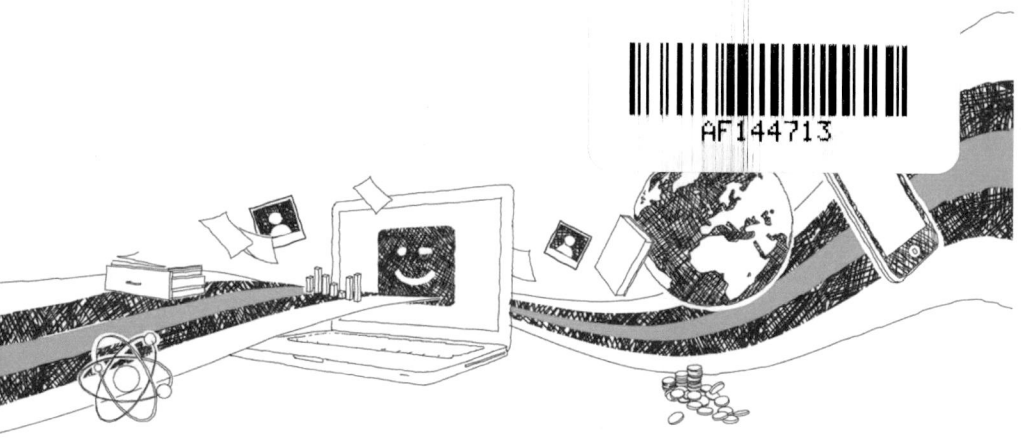
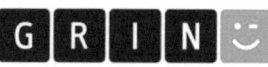

Bibliographic information published by the German National Library:

The German National Library lists this publication in the National Bibliography; detailed bibliographic data are available on the Internet at http://dnb.dnb.de .

Imprint:

Copyright © 2020 GRIN Verlag
Print and binding: Books on Demand GmbH, Norderstedt Germany
ISBN: 9783346238306

This book at GRIN:

https://www.grin.com/document/903467

Gizem Köprülülü Kücük, Nazli Irmak Giritlioglu

Cancer Development and Different Treatment Approaches

A Short Overview

GRIN Verlag

GRIN - Your knowledge has value

Since its foundation in 1998, GRIN has specialized in publishing academic texts by students, college teachers and other academics as e-book and printed book. The website www.grin.com is an ideal platform for presenting term papers, final papers, scientific essays, dissertations and specialist books.

CANCER DEVELOPMENT AND TREATMENT APPROACHES

GİZEM KÖPRÜLÜLÜ KÜÇÜK & NAZLI IRMAK GİRİTLİOĞLU

1. Cancer Development

Cancer is the uncontrolled division, proliferation, and accumulation of cells in an organism. It can affect a single organ as well as spread to distant organs and show its effect. Cancer has been a common problem in humans and animals throughout known history (Pavlopoulou A. et al., 2015). Cancer is a complex disease that occurs with uncontrolled division and proliferation of cells and under the influence of genetic and environmental conditions. Cancer is also a personal disease, although there are more than 100 known types of cancer and standard approaches have been developed for certain types of cancers (Fitzmaurice C. et al., 2015). It is not surprising that people have different responses to similar treatments since the DNA of any person in the world is not alike. With the advancement of technology, new treatment methods are being developed in addition to the treatments available today. In addition to the standard chemotherapy, radiotherapy and surgical methods, vaccines, biological, hormonal, targeted and gene therapies are increasingly being used. Although some standards have been determined, different approaches and treatments are applied for each type of cancer (Guo C., et al., 2013). The genes on the chromosomes are tightly packed, and physical or chemical changes on these genes can directly affect the cell's function. Although DNA repair systems try to restore the function of the gene due to damage to the gene, success is not always achieved. In this case, inadequate or incorrect production of proteins, which are the products of genes, disrupts cellular functions. Another factor that changes the function of the gene is epigenetic modifications such as methylation, acetylation, phosphorylation, ribosylation, which change the function of the gene without changing its structure. These modifications can only act on a specific site, or they may appear as regional deletions, insertions, or inversions that affect all or a large part of the chromosomes. Three gene groups are responsible for the formation of cancer. These are oncogenes, tumor suppressor genes, and DNA repair genes. Proto-oncogenes, which are normal genes that enable cell growth and differentiation, can become active and turn into oncogenes due to mutations, increased gene expression, gene duplications, and/or chromosomal rearrangements. Examples of the most known oncogenes are genes such as RAS, Erk, MYC. The gene groups that control the division and proliferation of the cell, initiate DNA repair in case of damage, and trigger apoptosis if the repair attempt fails, are called tumor suppressor genes. The most known and most studied of these is the TP53 gene. Deletions, point mutations, epigenetic silences, improper separation of chromosomes, and mitotic recombinations can lead to loss of function of the tumor suppressor gene, leading to loss of control in the cell cycle and carcinogenesis.

Cancer-causing agents are called carcinogens. These are examined in 3 groups: physical, chemical, and biological. Radiation, cigarette smoke, and viruses are examples of these carcinogens, respectively (Table 1) (Blackadar CB., 2016).

Table 1. Carcinogens and Cancer Types. When we look at the rates of development of cancer types, the most common type of cancer that causes death in both men and women is lung cancer. In the second place, prostate cancer in men and breast cancer in women (Siegel RL. et al., 2016).

Carcinogen	Type	Cancer
Chemical Carcinogen	Cigarette smoke	Lung Cancer
Biological Carcinogen	Human Papilloma Virus (HPV)	Cervical Cancer
Physical Carcinogen	UV	Skin Cancer

Cancer is responsible for 1 in 6 deaths globally. Tobacco using has approximately 22% rate which is the highest percentage of cancer deaths (https://www.who.int/news-room/fact-sheets/detail/cancer). The most common cancer types are lung and breast cancers worldwide. Respectively 2,093,876 and 2,088,849 cases were diagnosed in these cancer types in 2018. According to 2018 data, the most common cancer type among women is breast cancer and the most common cancer type among men is lung cancer (https://www.wcrf.org/dietandcancer/cancer-trends/worldwide-cancer-data) Common types of cancer types in both genders and separate genders are shown in Table 2 and Table 3.

2. Properties and Metabolism of Cancer Cells

Cancer cells are clever cells. They have their metabolism. Under normal conditions, when cells receive signals from the outer membrane, they grow and divide and multiply. The signals coming from outside enter into the cell, transferred to the nucleus and the process begins. Before the cell divides, it checks its surroundings and checks whether there are enough nutrients, whether there is room to grow, and begins to grow if conditions are favorable. They grow until they reach the predetermined height and number and stop growing as they touch each other. This is called contact inhibition (stop contact growth).

Table 2. Incidence of cancer types globally for both sexes in 2018 (https://www.wcrf.org/dietandcancer/cancer-trends/worldwide-cancer-data)

All cancers types	% of all cancer types (Excludes non-melanoma skin cancer)
Lung	12.3
Breast	12.3
Colorectal	10.6
Prostate	7.5
Stomach	6.1
Liver	5.0
Oesophagus	3.4
Cervix uteri	3.3
Thyroid	3.3
Bladder	3.2
Non-Hodgkin lymphoma	3.0
Pancreas	2.7
Leukemia	2.6
Kidney	2.4
Corpus uteri	2.2
Lip, oral cavity	2.1
Brain, central nervous system	1.7
Ovary	1.7
Melanoma of skin	1.7
Gallbladder	1.3
Larynx	1.0
Multiple myeloma	0.9
Nasopharynx	0.8
Oropharynx	0.5
Hypopharynx	0.5
Hodgkin lymphoma	0.5
Testis	0.4
Salivary glands	0.3
Anus	0.3
Vulva	0.3
Kaposi sarcoma	0.2
Penis	0.2
Mesothelioma	0.2
Vagina	0.1

Table 3: Top three cancer types and their number of cases in men and women according to 2018 data (https://www.wcrf.org/dietandcancer/cancer-trends/worldwide-cancer-data)

	Most common cancer types and case numbers		% of all cancer types
Men	Lung	1,368,524	15.5
	Prostate	1,276,106	14.5
	Colorectal	1,006,019	11.4
Women	Breast	2,088,849	25.4
	Colorectal	794,958	9.7
	Lung	725,352	8.8

If the DNA or one of the elements of the cell is damaged, the cells stop growing and dividing and pass to a phase called the G0 phase to be repaired. If the cell is repaired with the necessary arrangements here, it enters the circulation again and continues its life. However, if it is damaged beyond repair, it is sent to death programmatically through the mechanism called apoptosis, or the immune system cells destroy the damaged cell by eating it. Thus, transferring the damaged DNA to the next generations is prevented. Cancer cells have many features that normal cells do not have.

Receivers (receptors) on the cell surface receive signals more often

• It has its own signal systems that enable uncontrolled reproduction.

• It does not stop the division after contact with the next cell and continues to grow and multiply

• While healthy cells can use any type of food, cancer cells can only use glucose from glycolysis. They absorb sugar approximately 100 times more than normal cells and produce energy by producing lactate (Warburg effect).

• They can create new vascular systems by affecting the stroma around them to get the necessary nutrients and oxygen (neo-vascularization)

• Replicate and reproduce infinitely by fixing their telomeres or maintaining telomerase activity.

• They can enter the circulatory system and move to a distant place and start cancer in a new setting (metastasis)

• They can avoid apoptosis

• They are not genetically and epigenetically stable

Cancer cells are clever cells because they hold on to life with little oxygen, little food, resistance to harsh conditions, and turning these conditions in their favor over time. Cancer cells can be transformed over time, that is, deformed. While normal cells can grow and survive by clinging to a certain surface, cancer cells can live and grow and reproduce without holding anywhere. An abnormal cell occurs with the action of carcinogens from the normal cell. This cell divides to form a tumor mass. The resulting tumor mass needs food for its energy needs. They provide this nutrient requirement from glucose in our body. They form blood vessels branching out of our veins. This process is called angiogenesis. With these vascular networks, they use glucose in our blood as a source of energy to increase their reproduction. A cell that then leaves this tumor mass can pass to a different organ using the blood or lymph tract. We call this transfer metastasis. If these cancerous cells begin to spread to different regions in the organ where they first appeared, we call it an invasion (Figure 1).

Many types of cancer do not show symptoms at the beginning and it should be remembered that not all cancer types are the same. General symptoms, depending on the type of cancer, may vary. Therefore, the approach to each type of cancer is different. However, with early diagnosis, good care increases expected life expectancy and quality. Therefore, new methods are being tried. Although regular checks are important in the early diagnosis of cancer, many people have their checks after serious health problems. People with a family history of cancer should be more sensitive about routine checks. X-ray, blood tests, computed tomography scans, magnetic resonance imaging (MRI), endoscopy, and genetic imaging tests are tools that can be used in early diagnosis of cancer.

3. Cancer Treatment Approaches

Treatment approaches used in cancer treatment are radiotherapy, chemotherapy, and surgical methods. However, these methods, known as the gold standard, have advantages and disadvantages. Therefore, in addition to these conventional methods, various immunological and biological treatment methods are developed.

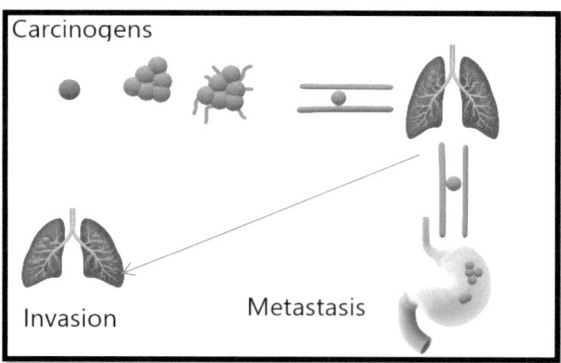

Figure 1. Cancer Pathway (Inspired by Kim et. al., 2009)

It is possible to make an early diagnosis with genetic tests to determine cancer susceptibility in individuals with a family history of cancer. In addition, the reasons behind the disease can be determined more precisely with these tests. Although useful information can be obtained thanks to these tests, it is possible that the person will never get the disease even though he has the gene that causes the disease.

3.1. Radiotherapy

Radiotherapy (RT) is a treatment method based on killing cancerous cells using ionizing rays. While it can be done by targeting only a certain part of the body, treatments targeting the whole body are also applied. The aim of radiotherapy is to provide protection of healthy tissues and risky organs while it gives the maximum dose to the tumor. RT is divided into two as external RT and brachytherapy, depending on how the radiation is applied to the patient. In external RT, radiation is applied to the patient at a certain distance with appropriate devices. Brachytherapy is the application of radiation by placing the radioactive source in or around the tumor. Devices used in RT also vary depending on these applications (Kinhikar RA. et al., 2014).

Different radiotherapy devices can be used in the treatment of radiotherapy depending on the general health of the patient, the type and stage of cancer (Varela G et al.,2016).
• The choice of the radiation source to be used is determined by the type of tumor, its location in the body, and especially its depth.

TrueBeam, Trilogy, Elekta Versa HD, and Linac devices are used during radiotherapy treatment.

Table 4. Examples of frequent tests depending on cancer types

Cancer Type	Test
Breast and over cancer	BRCA1-BRCA2
Breast, sarcoma, leukemia cancer	TP53
Over, colorectal, brain and endometrial cancer	MSH2, MLH1, MSH6
Colon, rectum, small intestine, stomach, skin cancer	APC
Eyes, bones and skin cancer	RB1

3.2. TrueBeam X

TrueBeam system, which is a new generation beam technology, is used in radiation oncology for irradiation of the tumor in every part of the body.

• TrueBeam has advantages such as robotic imaging, automatic patient positioning, motion management and dynamically synchronizing therapy. In addition, TrueBeam is often used for the treatment of tumors in hard-to-reach areas.

The biggest difference from other radiotherapy devices is the ability to increase the high dose rate. Thus, radiotherapy significantly reduces the session, duration, and number.

3.3. Trilogy

• Combining the features of all radiotherapy devices, Trilogy ensures that the correct intervention is performed in a shorter time and in the most appropriate amount.

• The uses of each of the methods used in the Trilogy are different; varies according to the structure of the tumor and the patient.

• Trilogy device can be examined in 3 different methods as IMRT, IGRT, SRT / SRC:

1. In the IMRT (Intensity Adjusted RT) method, the intensity of the radiation in the cancerous region is adjusted and the desired dose distribution is closest to the ideal. While high doses can be applied to the tumor, healthy tissues are also protected to the maximum.

2. In the IGRT (Imaging Guided RT) method, the patient can be visualized not only before the treatment but also during the treatment and the shifts in the area to be irradiated can be

prevented. In the IGRT method, the accuracy of the treatment area of the patients is certain with the imaging added to the device.

3. With the SRT / SRC method, spot irradiation can be performed on very small tumors of a millimeter level. With this irradiation performed as a point shot, a high dose of radiation is given to the tumor and healthy tissues are preserved (Chen H. et al., 2015).

3.4. Elekta Versa

• Elekta Versa provides the most accurate calculation of the doses given to the patient during radiotherapy.

In this way, damage to solid organs is prevented. Elekta Versa has a structure with 5 times less leakage dose permeability in linear accelerators.

• One of its biggest advantages is protecting healthy organs and minimizing the risk of secondary cancer formation.

• Elekta Versa shortens the treatment time compared to other devices.

3.5. Linac

• High energy x-rays and electron beams are obtained with this device.

• Linear accelerators usually have 2 x beam, 5-6 electron beam energy level. So different energy levels can be created in terms of usage.

• Linear accelerators have evolved over the years, while the energy of the resulting beam has increased, techniques have been developed that surround the tumor better and protect healthy tissues better.

3.6. Chemotherapy

Chemotherapy is a treatment method that aims to kill cancer cells using chemotherapeutic agents. Chemotherapy can be administered as neoadjuvant therapy or alone to reduce the size of the tumor before surgery. Drugs given during chemotherapy applications are alkylating agents, corticosteroids, anti-metabolites, anti-tumor antibiotics, mitotic inhibitors, and topoisomerase inhibitors. Alkylating agents are agents that suppress protein production by inhibiting the transcription of DNA (Patil Y. et al., 2016). If it enters the cell, the alkyl groups on the DNA are replaced by hydrogen atoms and show a carcinogenic effect. It has been shown that chemotherapy has been proven to be an effective treatment for cancer types such as Leukemia and lymphoma (Mian M. et al., 2016).

3.7. Surgery

Surgery is a common method for cancer therapy and it can bu used with radiotherapy and/or chemotherapy. Radiotherapy, which is applied before the surgical method, allows reducing the size of the tumor, while its application after surgery destroys cancer cells that may be left behind from the tumor tissue. It is very often used for the prevention of developing cancers, for prophylactic, taking a piece of tissue (biopsy), and for removing cancerous tissue/mass from the body in cases where there is no metastasis or spread. In cases where it is not possible to remove the mass without damaging other tissues, the surgeon may choose to shrink the mass with chemotherapy or radiotherapy before proceeding with the removal of a part of the mass. The surgical procedure can finally be used for the restoration and reconstruction of the damaged tissue/area. Apart from conventional techniques, laparoscopic surgery, using smaller probes or liquid nitrogen, which causes smaller scarring and complications by imaging the inside of the body with a special camera system, robotic surgery used in sensitive and hard-to-reach places, laser surgery using high-intensity rays. Many successful surgical procedures are frequently performed thanks to various techniques such as electrosurgery using high-frequency electric current.

3.8. Hormone Therapy

Hormones are proteins that are naturally produced in the body or chemical regulators that are given externally according to the need. These molecules enter the circulation and control the behavior of tissues and organs through endocrine signals. Hormones can be used as a medicine in cancer treatment. These are sex hormones commonly used in the treatment of prostate, breast, and endometrial cancers. These drugs prevent the hormone naturally produced by the body from binding to the cell and the growth of cancer cells.

3.9. Immunotherapy

The purpose of biological treatments is to treat cancer using biological substances. Monoclonal antibodies, cancer vaccines, anti-tumorigenic (inhibitors of cancer growth), antiangiogenic (inhibitors of blood vessels growth), interferons, interleukins, and gene therapy can be classified as subgroups of biological therapy.

Immunotherapy is carried out using the body's immune system's response to internal and external stimuli. Three main groups of molecules are frequently used in the treatment of cancer. These are cytokines, antibodies, and cells. The purpose of the treatment is to activate the immune system and attack cancer cells. This can be done using the body's own immune system or synthetic stimulants (monoclonal antibodies) (Grover NS. Et al., 2015).

Cancer vaccines are similar to conventional vaccines that stimulate the immune system and prevent disease by using attenuated molecules. The only difference is the targeting of cancer cells (Wei XX. et. al., 2015).

3.10. Gene Therapy

In classical gene therapies, genes are introduced into the cell directly or indirectly. This insertion process can be done outside the cell in laboratory conditions (ex vivo) or it can be done in vivo. In ex vivo transfer methods, cloned cells are inserted into the cells in the culture, and transferred to the patient after transfer by transfection. Autologous cells are often used to prevent the body from rejecting these new external cells. One of the major disadvantages of this method is the limited size of the transferred DNA fragments that can be inserted into the cell. In in vivo gene transfer, cloned cells are introduced directly into the patient's tissues. For this purpose, liposomes or viral vectors are used as carriers. Genes inserted after gene transfer either integrate into chromosomes or remain non-chromosome elements (episomes). The biggest advantage of inserting the gene into the chromosome is to make it permanent in the chromosome so that it can be used in hereditary treatments. However, integration in the wrong area is a common problem in this process because the genetic structure of people differs from each other. In such cases, this integration can lead to the death of the host cell, since the expression of the inserted gene will not be expressed (expression). The advantage of ex vivo transfer is that it can be chosen where the integration will be performed and the cells that have been successfully transfected can be transferred from the culture with higher success rates.

The aim of the treatment against cancer cells is to achieve high efficiency in a shorter time and to kill cancer cells in the shortest time. Thus, the need for recurring transfer in the long term will decrease. Structures that carry genes are called vectors. In general, two types of methods are used to insert the desired gene into the cell using the vector. The first is viral methods, and the other is non-viral (non-viral) methods. Gene therapy may fail because the immune system recognizes the vector as a foreign substance. Viral vectors: Viral vectors have a high transfer efficiency, but can only carry a limited size charge. If they are not properly modified, they can also infect the patient, since they are of viral origin. The most commonly used viral vectors are adeno-associated virus vectors (AAV), herpes simplex virus (HSV), vaccinia, retrovirus, and lentivirus vectors (Zabner J. et al.,1993).

REFERENCES

Blackadar CB. Historical review of the causes of cancer. World J Clin Oncol. 2016;7(1):54-86.

Chen H, Louie AV, Boldt RG, Rodrigues GB, Palma DA, Senan S. Quality of Life After Stereotactic Ablative Radiotherapy for EarlyStage Lung Cancer: A Systematic Review. Clin Lung Cancer. 2015 Dec 22. pii: S1525-7304(15)00303-4 9.

Fitzmaurice C, Dicker D, Pain A, Hamavid H, Moradi-Lakeh M, MacIntyre MF, Allen C ve ark. The Global Burden of Cancer 2013. JAMA Oncol. 2015;1(4):505-27. 2.

Grover NS, Park SI. Novel Targeted Agents in Hodgkin and NonHodgkin Lymphoma Therapy. Pharmaceuticals (Basel). 2015 Sep 17;8(3):607-36

Guo C, Manjili MH, Subjeck JR, Sarkar D, Fisher PB, Wang XY. Therapeutic cancer vaccines: past, present, and future. Adv Cancer Res. 2013; 119:421-75.

Kim, H. D., Youn, B., Kim, T. S., Kim, S. H., Shin, H. S., & Kim, J. (2009). Regulators affecting the metastasis suppressor activity of Nm23-H1. Molecular and Cellular Biochemistry. https://doi.org/10.1007/s11010-009-0109-2

Kinhikar RA, Pawar AB, Mahantshetty U, Murthy V, Dheshpande DD, Shrivastava SK. Rapid Arc, helical tomotherapy, sliding window intensity modulated radiotherapy and three dimensional conformal radiation for localized prostate cancer: a dosimetric comparison. J Cancer Res Ther. 2014 ;10(3):575-82.

Mian M, Tinelli M, DE March E, Turri G, Meneghini V, Pescosta N, Berno T ve ark. Bortezomib, Thalidomide and Lenalidomide: Have They Really Changed the Outcome of Multiple Myeloma? Anticancer Res. 2016;36(3):1059-65

Patil Y, Amitay Y, Ohana P, Shmeeda H, Gabizon A. Targeting of pegylated liposomal mitomycin-C prodrug to the folate receptor of cancer cells: Intracellular activation and enhanced cytotoxicity. J Control Release. 2016; 225:87-95.

Pavlopoulou A, Spandidos DA, Michalopoulos I. Human cancer databases (review). Oncol Rep. 2015 Jan;33(1):3-18.

Siegel RL, Miller KD, Jemal A. Cancer statistics, 2015. CA Cancer J Clin. 2015;65(1):5-29.

Varela G, Gómez-Hernández MT. Stereotactic ablative radiotherapy for early stage non-small cell lung cancer: a word of caution. Transl Lung Cancer Res. 2016 Feb;5(1):102-5.

Wei XX, Fong L, Small EJ. Prostate Cancer Immunotherapy with Sipuleucel-T: Current Standards and Future Directions. Expert Rev Vaccines. 2015;14(12):1529-41

Zabner J, Couture, LA, Gregory RJ, Graham SM, Smith AE, Welsh MJ. Adenovirus-mediated gene transfer transiently corrects the chloride transport defect in nasal epithelia of patients with cystic fibrosis. Cell. 1993;75(2):207-16

Internet References

Worldwide cancer data, reached on https://www.wcrf.org/dietandcancer/cancer-trends/worldwide-cancer-data, 21.06.2020.

Cancer, World Health Organization, reached on https://www.who.int/news-room/fact-sheets/detail/cancer, 21.06.2020.

YOUR KNOWLEDGE HAS VALUE

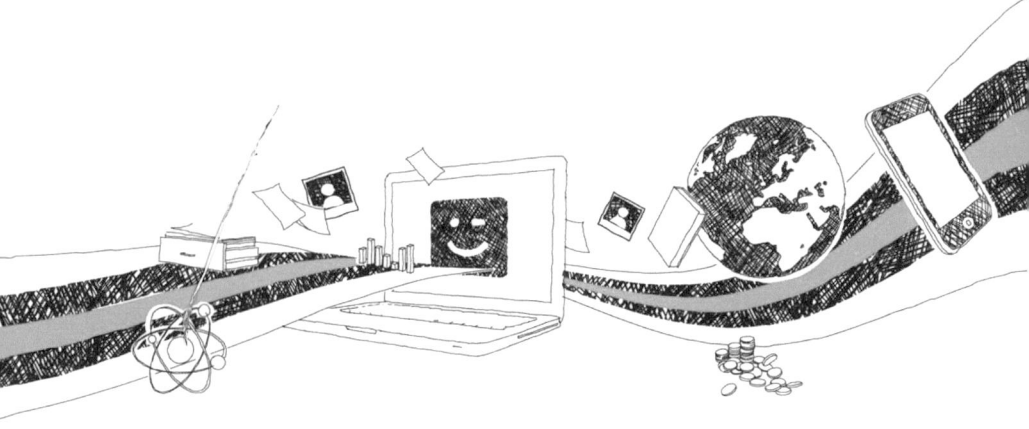

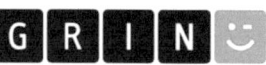